LIVING WITH DISEASE

ALZHEIMER'S DISEASE

BY BILL McAULIFFE

CREATIVE EDUCATION

Contents

Sandra Day O'Connor's husband

John had always been a joke-teller. But around the time he turned 60, he began forgetting the punch lines. "He thought maybe something was wrong, and so did I. And sure enough, it was," said O'Connor, the first woman to sit on the United States Supreme Court. Indeed, John O'Connor, an attorney, had Alzheimer's disease, which had begun to erode his memory, his intellect, and his personality. In time, Sandra's husband forgot her so thoroughly that when she went to visit him in a care center, they would chat as he held the hand of another woman at the center with whom he'd fallen in love. Remarkably, Sandra said she was happy her husband had found some joy. But her story also illustrates how this increasingly prevalent and incurable disease presents its victims and their loved ones with some of life's most difficult challenges.

Opposite page: Sandra Day O'Connor and her husband John at the Great Wall of China in 1987.

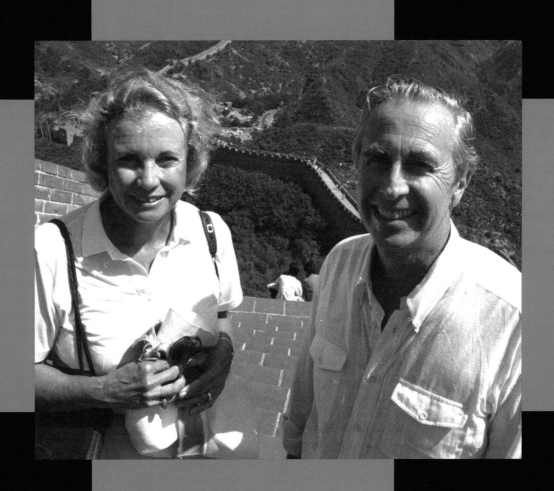

CHAPTER ONE

A "NEW" DISEASE

A little more than a century ago, people in the U.S. and Canada could expect to live about 47 years. Today, that's young. A baby born today can expect to celebrate 78 to 81 birthdays. A longer life span has allowed people to get to know their grandchildren and great-grandchildren better, to be more productive in their careers, to make more of a mark on their communities, and to pursue their personal interests more deeply. But it has also led to the **proliferation** of a devastating health threat: Alzheimer's disease.

Alzheimer's disease is a condition that affects older people almost exclusively, steadily destroying the physical structure of the brain and, with it, most of the person's unique human qualities. The disease robs its victims of their abilities to think and reason, to recognize loved ones, and even to perform such basic tasks as dressing and using the toilet. Over the course of sometimes 20 years or more, Alzheimer's can transform a patient's personality, making a previously sociable and happy person angry, frightened, and aggressive. Amid a fog of confusion, people with Alzheimer's frequently wander from home or from their care centers,

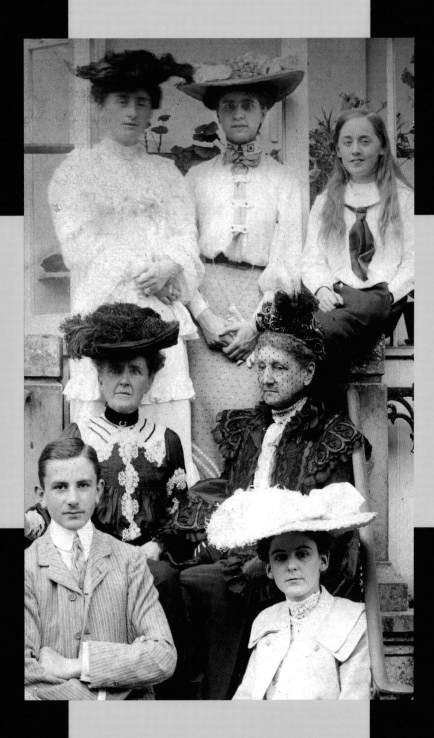

In the early 1900s, Alzheimer's disease was virtually unheard of because the average life span was much shorter than it is today.

often into dangerous situations. Slowly, they decline to an almost infantile condition, sometimes unable to speak or make sense of the world around them and completely dependent on others.

Alzheimer's disease is the most common form of dementia, a general decline in a person's **cognitive** abilities. Dementia, known in the past as senility, is characterized by memory loss, absent-mindedness, and confusion. Although the features of dementia are considered a normal part of aging, the symptoms of Alzheimer's disease are not. They are much more severe and caused by an ongoing physical deterioration of the brain. The disease affects more and more elderly people every year.

Alzheimer's disease almost always strikes people who are 65 or older, and because most people didn't live that long in the past, scientists of more than a century ago didn't study it. But in Germany in 1901, the family of a 51-year-old woman named Auguste Deter brought her to a psychiatric hospital with some baffling symptoms. She'd been having memory lapses, accusing her husband of spending time with other women, and having trouble speaking and understanding what was said to her. Her condition only got worse, until she died in 1906.

When psychiatrist Alois Alzheimer performed an **autopsy** and examined Deter's brain, he found that it had shrunk by about one-third,

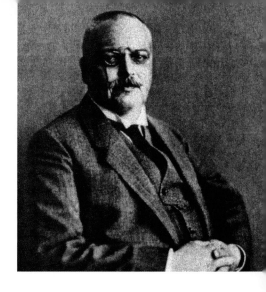

particularly the parts involved in thinking, memory, judgment, and speech. There were also unusual, dark clusters of material in the spaces between brain cells. He'd seen these clusters before, but only in the brains of much older people. Moreover, many of the remaining living cells contained strange, ropy tangles within them. He concluded that the abnormalities had caused Deter's disorder and her death, and in 1906, he gave a lecture on the subject that would later make him famous.

Alzheimer himself saw only two cases of Alzheimer's disease in his career. But it's now estimated that 5.3 million people in the U.S. have Alzheimer's disease to one degree or another, with another 500,000 people suffering from the disease in Canada. Due to an aging population and better awareness of the disease, those numbers are expected to nearly triple by 2050. Worldwide, about 35 million people have Alzheimer's disease. Unless ways are found to prevent, stall, or cure the disease, the global number is expected to multiply to more than 115 million by 2050.

Alzheimer's disease caused nearly 75,000 deaths in the U.S. in 2007. That made it the sixth-leading cause of death. The death rate from Alzheimer's is far lower than from heart disease and cancer. Even so, over recent decades it has claimed some of the world's most accomplished

German psychiatrist
Alois Alzheimer,
pictured around 1914.

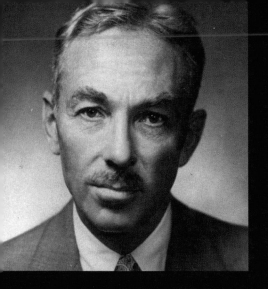

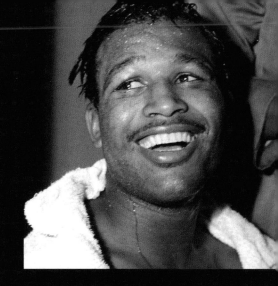

Only about 0.1 percent of people in the U.S. younger than 65 have Alzheimer's. About 13 percent of American men and women over the age of 65 have been diagnosed with the disease. But nearly half of those 85 and older are living with it.

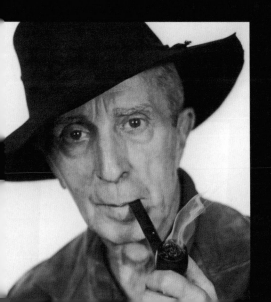

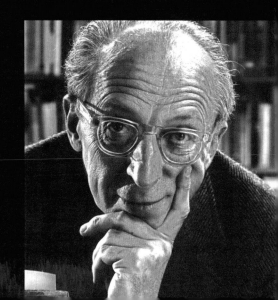

people. Essayist and author E. B. White, who wrote *Charlotte's Web*, died of it at age 86. So did composer Aaron Copland, at age 90; artist Norman Rockwell, at 84; and boxing champion Sugar Ray Robinson, at 67.

U.S. president Ronald Reagan focused attention on the disease in 1983 by declaring November to be National Alzheimer's Disease Month. In 1994, 5 years after leaving office, Reagan himself, then 82, was diagnosed with Alzheimer's. He died of its effects in June 2004.

The attention brought to Alzheimer's by Reagan's illness and the increasingly aging U.S. population helped focus researchers' energy on the disease. In fact, according to the Alzheimer's Association, most of what is known about Alzheimer's today has been learned since 1990. Significant strides have been made in understanding the causes of Alzheimer's disease, how it differs from other forms of age-related mental deterioration, and how victims and their loved ones can cope with it.

Alzheimer's disease is not contagious, but it is often **hereditary**. About 30 percent of people with Alzheimer's disease have a parent or grandparent who had the disease, and people whose mother and father both had Alzheimer's have a notably increased risk of getting it themselves. Younger-onset Alzheimer's occurs in people under the age of 65

Opposite page, clockwise from left: E. B. White, Sugar Ray Robinson, Aaron Copland, and Norman Rockwell.

11

Alzheimer's Strikes a President

After completing a two-term presidency (1981–89), Ronald Reagan stayed busy answering letters, making a few public appearances, and corresponding with other former presidents. But in 1993, Reagan was in Chicago and told his wife, Nancy, that he couldn't remember where he was. At a dinner for the former prime minister of Great Britain, he repeated a paragraph in his speech without knowing it. In 1994, doctors told Reagan he had Alzheimer's disease, and a year later, he bade a public farewell to the American people. Many suspected that Reagan's Alzheimer's stemmed from hitting his head on a rock after falling from a horse in 1989, but that connection was never proven. In 1995, the Reagans joined with the Alzheimer's Association to establish the Ronald and Nancy Reagan Research Institute, helping spur new developments in understanding the disease. The former president died in 2004 at the age of 93.

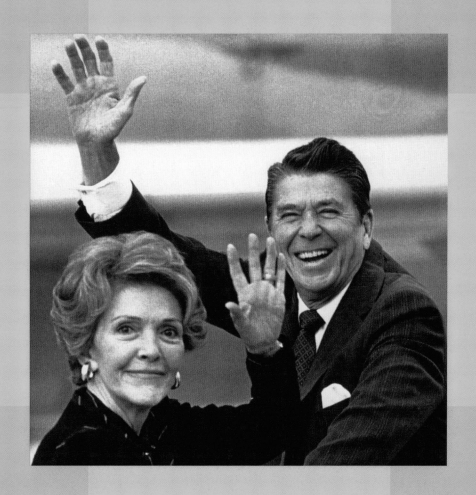

President-elect Ronald Reagan and his wife, Nancy, waving to bystanders in November 1980.

and affects roughly 500,000 Americans. Getting the disease in one's 30s, 40s, or 50s is linked even more closely to hereditable factors.

Still, researchers continue to look for causes of the disease far beyond family history. Age is the most common risk factor for Alzheimer's disease. High blood pressure is also suspected of being linked to Alzheimer's. So is experience with depression. Women get Alzheimer's more frequently than men, in part because they generally live longer. But other than that, no one really knows why some people get Alzheimer's disease and others don't.

Some studies have found that, among people with Alzheimer's, Hispanics and African Americans tend to be diagnosed at younger ages than whites. Researchers have also investigated possible links to smoking and exposure to aluminum, glues, pesticides, fertilizers, and even **electromagnetic fields**, but they haven't found clear evidence that any of these environmental factors cause Alzheimer's. Some researchers believe that other factors, such as educational level, diet, and even exercise—both physical and mental—might play a role in the development or prevention of the disease. In an aging society, finding the causes and possible treatments for Alzheimer's disease is an urgent challenge.

Alzheimer's disease killed nearly 23 out of every 100,000 people in the U.S. in 2007. That is a lower death rate than for heart disease (191), cancer (178), high blood pressure and related diseases (42), respiratory diseases (41), and accidents (38), but higher than for influenza and pneumonia (16).

CHAPTER TWO

BRAIN DETERIORATION

The human brain contains about

100 billion **neurons**, or nerve cells. The neurons have long tentacles that connect with each other at more than 100 trillion points to form a network that is often referred to as the "neuron forest." The neuron forest carries signals in the form of tiny electrical impulses. Chemicals called neurotransmitters help transmit the signals from neuron to neuron. The brain translates these signals into sensations, thinking, memory, movement, and emotions.

Alzheimer's disease represents the widespread destruction of this system, as brain cells die and signals between neurons are interrupted. The destruction is caused by a buildup of defective **proteins** in the brain. These proteins, which are produced by the body itself, can sometimes form materials that block signal pathways in the brain. Most often, they begin to disrupt the neuron communication system in the hippocampus, an area at the center of the brain. If the brain were a computer, the hippocampus would be its hard drive, where memory is generated. That's why memory loss is one of the first signs of Alzheimer's disease.

Every neuron has a cell body that contains a nucleus at its center.

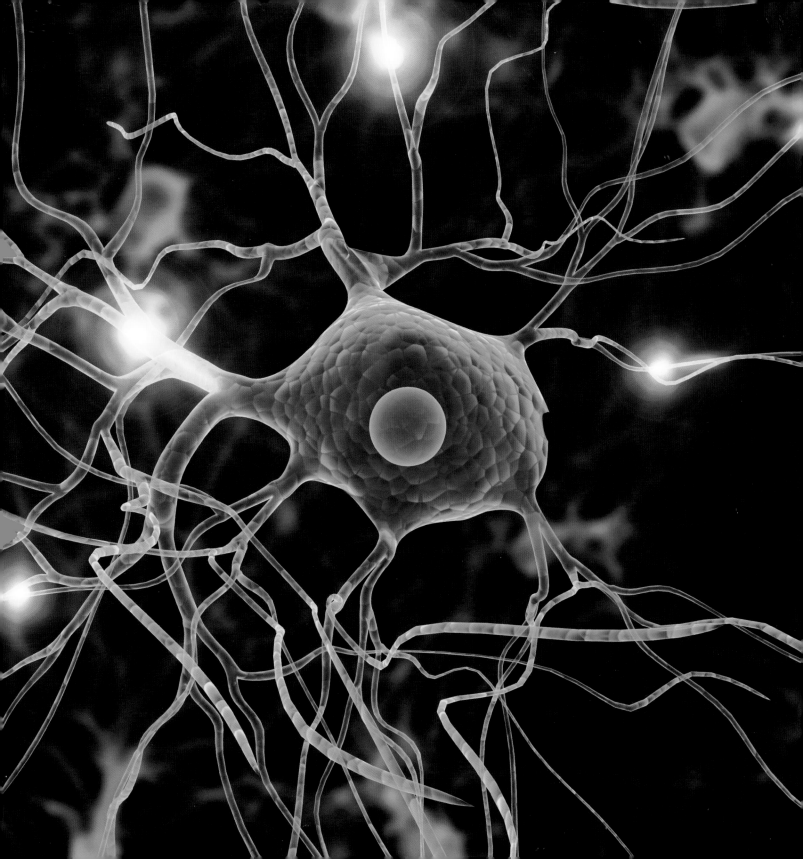

But the deterioration then spreads outward to all regions of the brain, undermining all of a person's intellectual and emotional capacity, as well as physical skills. One researcher called the accumulation of the defective proteins "a weapon of mass destruction" in the brain.

Scientists have further zeroed in on interactions between certain proteins and **enzymes** in the brain as a possible source of the signal-blocking materials. A substance called the amyloid precursor protein, which plays a role in the growth and survival of neurons, sticks through a cell's fatty **membrane** like whiskers. Different types of enzymes are supposed to clip off the proteins on the outside of the cell membrane. After they have been clipped off, the protein fragments usually dissolve. But when certain enzymes do the trimming, the fragments are longer and don't dissolve as readily. One such fragment, called beta-amyloid 42, clusters with other fragments to form plaques—abnormal, dense collections of proteins between neurons that interfere with cell-to-cell signaling. First noticed as dark clusters by Alzheimer himself in the brain of Auguste Deter, plaques are commonly found in the brains of Alzheimer's patients. Meanwhile, a protein called tau, which transports nutrients through healthy cells in a straight line, can collapse into tangles within cells. Eventually, a cell's

Amyloid plaques are also known as senile (for "old age") or dendritic (meaning "branched") plaques.

Naming Rights

Alois Alzheimer entered medical practice as an expert on earwax. But before long he turned his attention to mental illness. Born in 1864 in Bavaria (a region in southern Germany), Alzheimer earned his medical degree in 1887 and the next year joined the staff of a mental asylum. His identification in 1906 of irregularities in the brain of a woman who died after a long mental decline distinguished the condition from simple aging and remains the standard for the diagnosis of Alzheimer's disease. In 1903, Alzheimer established a research laboratory at the Royal Psychiatric Hospital in Munich, Germany. Assistants knew him for the cigars he smoked continually in the laboratory classrooms, but his fellow scientists knew him for his studies of brain changes associated with several physical diseases, including Alzheimer's. He died of a heart complication in 1915 at the age of 51.

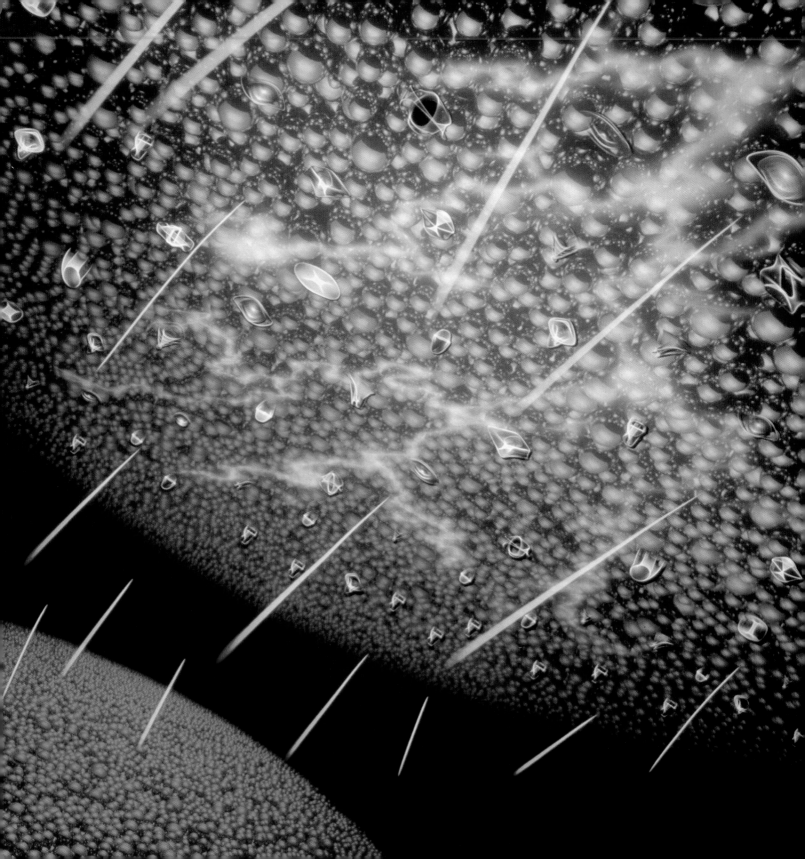

transport system disintegrates, and when nutrients can no longer travel through the cell, the cell dies. The tangles, which Alzheimer also noted, are another emblem of the disease.

A class of proteins known as apolipoprotein E, which controls how blood **cholesterol** is carried through the body, may also play a role in plaque formation. The APOE **gene** makes apolipoprotein E, and there are at least three alleles, or forms, of the gene. One of them (E4) increases the amount of beta-amyloid 42 in the brain, or at least is not as effective as the normal gene is in dissolving the plaque-forming substance. Inheriting this form of the gene increases one's chances of developing Alzheimer's.

Despite their understanding of the complex mechanics of Alzheimer's, doctors most often diagnose the disease based on what a patient doesn't have. All other possible causes of symptoms must be ruled out before a patient is determined to be suffering from Alzheimer's. For example, symptoms such as memory loss and confusion might also be caused by depression, stroke, a brain tumor, drug or alcohol use, or a condition called mild cognitive impairment, a form of dementia that resembles Alzheimer's. A person with mild cognitive impairment might have lost some memory but would have retained her ability to communicate sensibly and to understand others.

Certain proteins help nerve cells communicate with each other through electrical charges.

In attempting to determine whether or not a person suffers from Alzheimer's, doctors might also test her sense of smell. In the early stages of the disease, a patient can't distinguish between many smells and, for reasons that are unclear, loses the ability to detect the scents of strawberry, smoke, and soap. Later, she loses the ability to smell at all. This is because Alzheimer's destroys cells in the region of the brain where the sense of smell is located.

Most often, however, it is not the sense of smell but assessments by psychologists, social workers, and **neurologists** that are used to determine whether a person has Alzheimer's. A patient is often asked basic questions to determine her level of awareness, such as whether she knows where she is or what year it is. Then she might be asked to copy a geometric pattern, count backwards, or spell a familiar word backwards. A patient might also be asked to repeat a sequence of three words that she had been told to remember minutes before. If she has trouble responding, jumbles or struggles with words, or can't understand what numbers represent—an indication that she has lost some or all of the ability to think **abstractly**—that might support a diagnosis of Alzheimer's disease. In addition, the symptoms must be causing problems in the patient's everyday life and relationships and be getting progressively worse to indicate the presence of Alzheimer's disease.

Because they tend to live longer, women are nearly twice as likely as men to develop Alzheimer's disease. The disease can be expected to be diagnosed in about 1 of every 6 women and 1 of every 10 men age 55 and over in their remaining lifetimes.

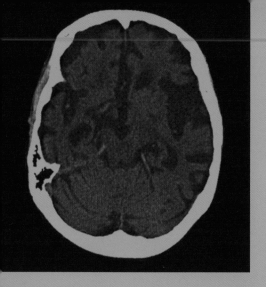

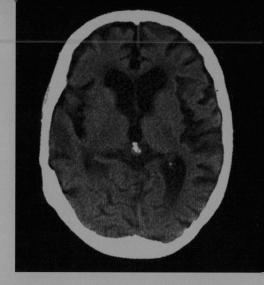

Medicare, the U.S. government's health insurance for people over the age of 65, spends 3 times more on care for patients with Alzheimer's disease than it pays for other patients. From 2005 to 2015, the amount it spends is expected to double, to $189 billion.

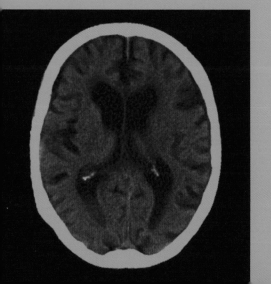

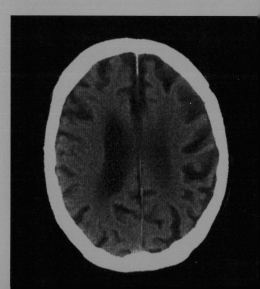

If the psychological or cognitive tests are inconclusive, or if doctors want to determine how far physical brain damage has progressed, a patient might undergo testing by sophisticated scanning devices. A computerized tomography (CT) scan involves a series of rotating X-rays, which generate images of the brain from numerous angles. In some cases, it can provide detailed glimpses of small parts of the brain, such as the hippocampus, where Alzheimer's frequently begins. A CT scan can also rule out other causes of cognitive loss by finding evidence of strokes or brain tumors. A magnetic resonance imaging (MRI) device uses radio waves and magnetic fields to detect small energy signals being emitted by **atoms** in brain tissues and is good at measuring the volume, or size, of the brain. A positron emission tomography (PET) scan measures emissions given off from injected **radioactive** material. It can map how a person's brain responds to music, writing, or conversation. Researchers have also recently used PET scans to determine where plaques are forming in people's brains. In addition, the scans can detect how the brain is using the sugar glucose, which is significant because diseased brains process glucose less effectively than do healthy brains.

The brain of an Alzheimer's patient can be visually examined by using CT scans.

CHAPTER THREE

THE CHALLENGE OF ALZHEIMER'S

A person diagnosed with Alzheimer's disease will fall into one of three stages of the disease: mild, moderate, or severe. A person with mild Alzheimer's has already suffered damage in the parts of the brain that affect memory, learning, thinking, and planning. He forgets recent events, struggles to remember and use well-known words, and asks the same question repeatedly. He might show signs of depression, which is regarded as both a symptom and a possible trigger of Alzheimer's. He can't follow a familiar recipe and often misplaces things in strange places—putting the television remote control in the refrigerator, for example. With mild Alzheimer's, a person might have a hard time understanding what's said to him. He might stop caring about dressing right, become increasingly anxious about future events or changes in routine, and act discourteously to other people. If he had been an outgoing, sociable person, he might become quiet and withdrawn. He might get lost driving in a familiar neighborhood. Frequently, his eyes might appear completely vacant, without any apparent thought or recognition.

Alzheimer's may be most frequently diagnosed in its moderate stage because symptoms become much more obvious than during the mild stage.

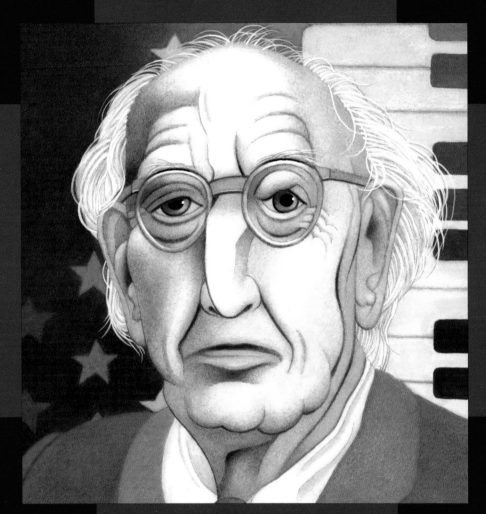

Aaron Copland composed the majority of his works before the 1980s, when his health declined due to Alzheimer's.

A Star Eclipsed

Rita Hayworth was one of Hollywood's brightest stars in the 1940s and '50s. The beautiful actress and dancer was famous the world over; during World War II, her pictures were common features in military housing units and ships. But in 1962, while trying to launch a career in stage acting, Hayworth pulled out of a play, unable to memorize her lines. She continued to act in movies until 1972, when she was 54, but became increasingly temperamental and irrational. Many blamed Hayworth's personality changes on heavy drinking, but in 1980, she was diagnosed with Alzheimer's disease. She died in 1987. During Hayworth's last years, her daughter, Princess Yasmin Aga Khan, publicized her mother's illness. Since 1985, Princess Yasmin has held exclusive, formal dinner dances named for her mother in New York, Chicago, and Dallas. The annual Rita Hayworth Galas have raised more than $53 million for the Alzheimer's Association.

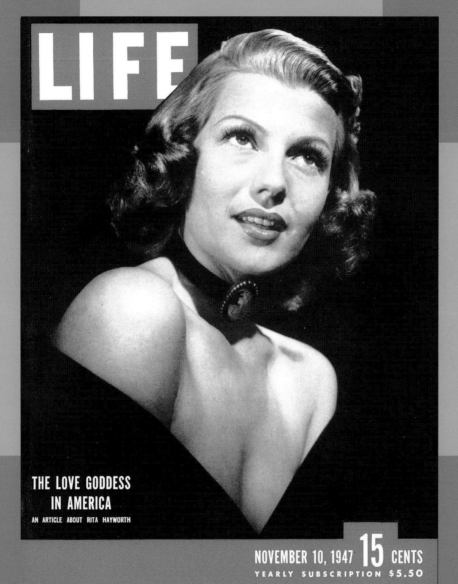

LIFE

THE LOVE GODDESS
IN AMERICA
AN ARTICLE ABOUT RITA HAYWORTH

NOVEMBER 10, 1947 **15** CENTS
YEARLY SUBSCRIPTION $5.50

Rita Hayworth made
the cover of *Life* in
November 1947.

(That may be one reason for the common claim that medical professionals can diagnose Alzheimer's disease with 90 percent accuracy.) People with moderate Alzheimer's often forget to turn off appliances or take their medications. They start to lose the ability to use utensils or tie shoelaces. At this stage, what might have seemed like old-age crabbiness often worsens into aggression, angry outbursts, swearing, or other behavior that's inappropriate in public. People with moderate Alzheimer's might also begin to experience **hallucinations** or become suspicious of others and be unable to reason or make sound decisions.

A person with severe Alzheimer's has little or no memory and cannot care for herself. She shows little emotion, doesn't recognize loved ones, and might not even recognize herself in the mirror. Because she has lost much of her ability to chew and swallow, the patient with severe Alzheimer's becomes weak and vulnerable to infections, falling into a final decline and death. On average, a person will live 4 to 8 years after being diagnosed with Alzheimer's, although some people live 20 or more years with the disease.

Several drugs have been approved to treat people with Alzheimer's. The drugs do not cure the disease, but they can slow its progress and ease its symptoms. When Alzheimer's disease damages or destroys brain cells, it also reduces the number of neurotransmitters in the brain. Several drugs are designed to slow the loss of neurotransmitters in surviving cells. Others remove substances

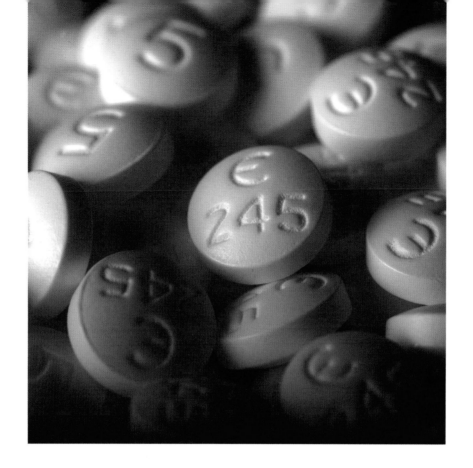

Donepezil, prescribed under such brand names as Aricept, can be an effective Alzheimer's treatment.

that block communications between neurons. Many Alzheimer's drugs have been shown to slow the pace of loss of memory, learning ability, and language skills. Among these are donepezil, which is prescribed most often to treat mild to moderate stages of Alzheimer's, along with galantamine and rivastigmine. A drug called memantine helps slow memory loss by regulating the activity of the neurotransmitter glutamate. It has been approved for use in moderate to severe cases of Alzheimer's disease.

Researchers are also trying to refine drugs that can alter some of the difficult behavior that comes with Alzheimer's. Antidepressants are used to fight low moods and irritability. Other drugs, called **anxiolytics**, work against anxiety, restlessness, loud outbursts, and resistant behavior. **Antipsychotic** drugs can reduce hallucinations, **delusions**, aggression, agitation, hostility, and uncooperativeness. However, some of these drugs can have severe side effects, including an increased risk of stroke. Or they can backfire and make the patient's symptoms worse. Medical professionals prescribe them only if the patient is a danger to himself or others.

Even with the availability of treatments, a diagnosis of Alzheimer's frequently devastates patients and their families. Patients often become depressed. This can complicate their situation, since they may find themselves unable to describe their feelings, which also tend to change more frequently than in depressed people who don't have Alzheimer's disease.

While the effects of Alzheimer's are devastating to its victims, the impact is twofold on their family members, who make up a fraction of the 50 million unpaid caregivers in the U.S. About 7 out of 10 people with Alzheimer's disease live at home, and as a patient loses her memory, constantly repeats herself, or gets uncharacteristically angry, family members may themselves get frustrated and annoyed. But the demands increase as the disease progresses. The patient may need her clothes laid out for her in the morning, then someone may have to remind her to put them on. She might need to be bathed and might need her hair brushed because she can't do such tasks herself or doesn't remember how

About 500,000 Canadians have Alzheimer's disease. Of those, nearly three-quarters are women. About 1 in 11 Canadians over the age of 65 has the disease, compared with 1 in 8 Americans in that age group. Canada expects to see as many as 1.1 million cases within a generation.

Care for Alzheimer's patients in the U.S. costs $172 billion per year. That doesn't account for the 10.9 million unpaid spouses, adult children, and others providing nearly 12.5 billion hours of care worth an estimated $144 billion. The comparable figures for Canada are 600,000 people providing $5 billion worth of care.

or why she should. Someone will need to take her to the bathroom during the night, and during the day someone will need to check on her, making sure, for example, that she hasn't left the stove on. Someone will need to make sure she hasn't wandered out the door. Even basic conversation can be troublesome, because a person with Alzheimer's can be argumentative.

Caregivers frequently fall into depression themselves as they find their own lives controlled by the needs of the Alzheimer's patient, usually a parent or spouse. They find they don't have time for friends anymore and that friends start avoiding them anyway because of their loved one's behavior. Money becomes a constant worry; drugs and extra help can be expensive, and caregivers often have to cut back on their own work or quit entirely. Children caring for parents with Alzheimer's frequently feel as if they've switched roles, and spouses often feel abandoned by their lifelong partners.

One way many people who care for someone with Alzheimer's can cope with the challenges is by seeking help from others. Many caregivers find it helpful to join a support group. As the disease progresses, many patients will need regular visits from a nurse or other professional who can administer medications. In any case, people with Alzheimer's will almost always reach a point where they will need round-the-clock skilled medical care, which likely means moving them into a nursing home.

CHAPTER FOUR

RESEARCH: GAINS AND SETBACKS

As is common with medical research,

investigating Alzheimer's disease has required a combination of tireless examination of tissues and cells, studies and comparisons of patients and groups, work with laboratory animals, collections of personal and family histories, and the use of advanced diagnostic machinery. Although research has quickly become a multibillion-dollar industry in the U.S., breakthroughs have been few. Indeed, much is still unknown about the causes of Alzheimer's. And because of that, there is still no cure.

But considering the high emotional and financial costs of Alzheimer's disease, researchers are exploring how new drugs and alternative treatments might be used to delay the onset of Alzheimer's, or at least ease some of its symptoms. Since the first drug for Alzheimer's treatment, called tacrine, was approved for use in the U.S. in 1993, only a handful of others have been developed. And there have been many frustrations. Tacrine itself was soon linked to liver damage in patients who took it and is rarely prescribed today. In addition, the first **vaccine** to offer some hope as a weapon against Alzheimer's was abandoned by researchers in 2005 after it was found that the immune response

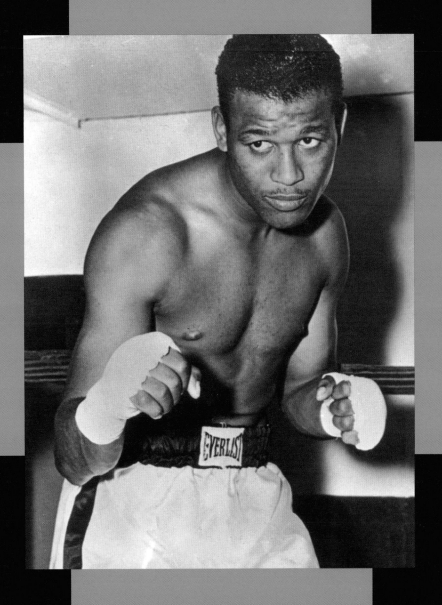

Six-time world champion boxer Sugar Ray Robinson died before much was known about Alzheimer's treatments.

Six states in the western U.S. are expected to see twice the number of people with Alzheimer's in 2025 as there were in 2000. In Alaska, Utah, Colorado, Wyoming, Idaho, and Nevada, the percentage of the population 65 and older is expected to increase faster than anywhere else in the country.

it provoked created inflammation in patients' brains. In 2010, latrepirdine, a drug that had earlier seemed to improve cognitive function and behavior in Alzheimer's patients, failed to show the same benefit in a trial.

Along with prescription drugs, research has also focused on vitamins and even the common anti-inflammatory drug ibuprofen, but their impact on Alzheimer's has been contradictory. Similarly, the natural tree extract ginkgo biloba, long believed to help improve memory, has been approved as an Alzheimer's treatment in Germany, but recent U.S. tests showed it had little value for Alzheimer's patients.

As with other diseases, research has shown that a healthy diet, regular exercise, sociability, and minimum alcohol intake all seem to help hold off Alzheimer's. Researchers have also been encouraged to find that caffeine, a key ingredient in coffee, has reversed memory loss in mice that have been bred to develop Alzheimer's disease. Caffeine also reduced the occurrence of beta-amyloid in the lab animals' bloodstreams.

In addition to looking for ways to slow or stop Alzheimer's and its symptoms, researchers continue to seek a better understanding of its causes. It's now believed that the formation of plaques between neurons and the collapse of tau proteins into tangles within neurons—the classic identifiers of Alzheimer's disease—sometimes begins 20 years before patients show symptoms of the disease. Dr. Zaven Khachaturian, the former director of Alzheimer's research at the National Institutes of Health, has even suggested that Alzheimer's may in fact not be an old person's disease, since so many of its suspected causes are present in patients many years before the first symptoms appear.

Researchers continue to search for a possible genetic link to Alzheimer's. But so far, only a few forms of the more than 30,000 genes per cell in the human body—including APOE—have been connected with Alzheimer's. In 2009, after examining the genes of 16,000 people, researchers led by the British Medical Research Council announced that they had identified **mutated** forms of 3 other genes that might be related to the onset of Alzheimer's. Like APOE, the genes are supposed to clear plaque-producing proteins from the brain, but their mutated forms fail to do this. The identification of the gene mutations was the first such breakthrough in Alzheimer's-related genetic research in 16 years. Identifying specific genes linked to Alzheimer's disease can help researchers target them and even begin trying to fix the genes in people who carry the mutant forms before they show symptoms.

Personal studies have also proven valuable in determining the risk factors that might lead to Alzheimer's disease. Beginning in 1986, **epidemiologist** David Snowdon examined decades' worth of medical histories of 678 nuns belonging to the School Sisters of Notre Dame. The nuns were considered a

A 106-year-old participant in the Nun Study shares a laugh with researcher David Snowdon in 2001.

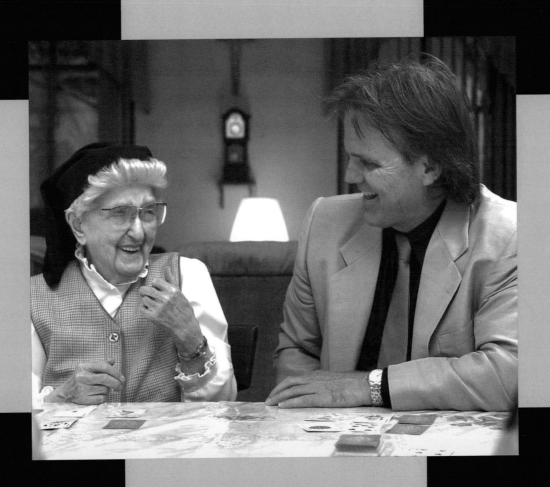

An Award for Research

The Potamkin Prize is the highest distinction given for research into Alzheimer's disease and related forms of dementia. Considered the Nobel Prize of dementia research, the $100,000 award was founded in 1988 by the family of Luba Potamkin, a television spokeswoman for the family's Cadillac car dealerships on the East Coast. She was diagnosed with Alzheimer's in 1978 and died in 1994. The prize is administered by the American Academy of Neurology and is awarded annually. Recipients have explored the development of Alzheimer's disease in mice, advanced understanding of the disease's early stages, and identified drugs that might target plaques and tangles in the brain. The award also recognizes significant research into Pick's disease, a rare and related form of dementia from which Luba Potamkin was later found to have died. Fifty-one scientists from around the world had won or shared the prize through 2010.

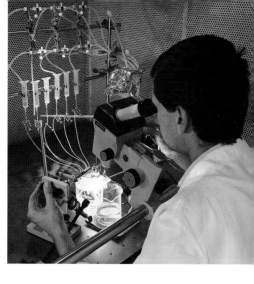

valuable group for research because they had had similar life-styles and lived in the same environment for almost their entire adult lives. Moreover, they'd kept writings going back to the days they'd entered the convent as 22-year-olds, and all participants agreed to donate their brains to the study (upon their death) as well.

In reading the nuns' youthful writings, Snowdon determined that the quality of a nun's writing as a young girl was a powerful predictor of whether or not she would contract Alzheimer's later in life. Writing that was less rich with ideas or showed less complex sentence structure was often the work of women who many years later developed Alzheimer's disease. Writing with more ideas and complex grammar, indicating a high-functioning memory, was done by women who later died without Alzheimer's. Snowdon was able to link the poorer writing with Alzheimer's victims with better than 85 percent accuracy. He also found that nuns who did not develop Alzheimer's disease shared another trait: having a positive or optimistic attitude through much of their lives.

The study, which was ongoing as of 2011, prompted further research into whether treatments could be prescribed for people who might be prone to Alzheimer's disease. But it also put a spotlight on how a mind's own nimbleness could help protect people from Alzheimer's. Other studies have suggested that

Researchers can study brains affected by Alzheimer's by looking at small sections under a microscope.

intellectual challenges such as reading, doing crossword puzzles, and playing a musical instrument reduce the risk of dementia. That's in part because neurons that are not stimulated die more quickly than others. But the fact that highly accomplished and creative people, such as President Reagan and Aaron Copland, have succumbed to the disease indicates how formidable—and puzzling—Alzheimer's continues to be.

Since Alois Alzheimer's name was first linked to the disease in 1907, Alzheimer's physical symptoms and effects on patients' lives have been clearly defined. But why the brain decay develops and the disease seems to affect the elderly almost exclusively remain mysteries. Meanwhile, living with Alzheimer's continues to be a sad and difficult challenge for both patients and their caretakers. Although patients become childlike, Alzheimer's is the opposite of childhood. It is a regression of unlearning and becoming less aware, less skilled, and less involved. Fortunately, new research offers hope of slowing that course—and maybe, someday, even preventing it.

A woman diagnosed with Alzheimer's desease at age 70 can expect to live about 8 more years, while a 70-year-old woman without the disease could expect to live twice that long. For men, life expectancy is 4.4 years for 70-year-olds diagnosed with Alzheimer's and 9.3 years for those without it.

GLOSSARY

abstractly: dealing with a subject only in the mind or through symbols or theories

antipsychotic: used to combat severe mental disorders characterized by a loss of contact with reality and often featuring delusions or hallucinations

anxiolytics: drugs that reduce anxiety or extreme fear

atoms: the smallest particles of an element that can exist alone

autopsy: an examination of a body's vital organs after death to determine the cause of death

cholesterol: a soft, waxy substance found in the bloodstream and all cells that is used to help digest fats and strengthen cell membranes; it can cause heart problems when it builds up in the blood

cognitive: having to do with the processes of thinking, learning, knowing, judging, and being aware

delusions: false beliefs regarding oneself or others that persist despite facts

electromagnetic fields: areas of energy surrounding electrical devices, such as power lines, antennae, electric power tools, lights, and appliances

enzymes: proteins that trigger chemical reactions in the body

epidemiologist: a person who studies the distribution and prevalence of diseases

gene: the basic unit of instruction in a cell, which controls a person's physical traits and passes characteristics from parents to offspring

hallucinations: perceptions of objects, sights, or sounds that do not exist

hereditary: passed on from parents to children through the genes

membrane: a thin, flexible layer that surrounds a cell and its components

mutated: changed in a relatively permanent way; a gene mutation results in a new characteristic or function in a cell

neurologists: physicians skilled in the diagnosis and treatment of diseases of the nervous system, including the brain

neurons: nerve cells capable of receiving electrical impulses or chemical signals from one cell and transmitting them to another

proliferation: a rapid increase

proteins: complex structures that are the basic components of all living cells

radioactive: relating to the spontaneous emission of energetic particles (such as electrons) as an atom decays

vaccine: a substance given in a shot or by mouth that helps the immune system form antibodies (disease-fighting proteins) to fight off a specific disease

BIBLIOGRAPHY

Alzheimer's Association National Office. "Alzheimer's Facts and Figures." Alzheimer's Association. http://www.alz.org/alzheimers_disease_facts_figures.asp.

Gruetzner, Howard. *Alzheimer's: A Caregiver's Guide and Sourcebook*. New York: John Wiley & Sons, 2001.

Hogan, Victoria. "Role Change Experienced by Family Caregivers of Adults with Alzheimer's Disease: Implications for Occupational Therapy." *Physical and Occupational Therapy in Geriatrics* 22, no. 1. (2004): 21–43.

Molloy, William, and Paul Caldwell. *Alzheimer's Disease: Everything You Need to Know*. Buffalo, N.Y.: Firefly Books, 2003.

Petersen, Ronald, ed. *Mayo Clinic on Alzheimer's Disease*. Rochester, Minn.: Mayo Clinic, 2002.

Shankle, William Rodman, and Daniel Amen. *Preventing Alzheimer's: Prevent, Detect, Diagnose, Treat, and Even Halt Alzheimer's Disease and Other Causes of Memory Loss*. New York: G. P. Putnam's Sons, 2004.

Xu, Jiaquan, Kenneth Kochanek, and Betzaida Tejada-Vera. "Deaths: Preliminary Data for 2007." *National Vital Statistics Reports* 58, no. 1. (August 19, 2009): 5.

Young, Ellen P. *Between Two Worlds: Special Moments of Alzheimer's & Dementia*. Amherst, N.Y.: Prometheus Books, 1999.

FURTHER READING

Brill, Marlene Targ. *Alzheimer's Disease*. New York: Benchmark Books, 2005.

Landau, Elaine. *Alzheimer's Disease: A Forgotten Life*. New York: Franklin Watts, 2005.

McGuigan, Jim. *Alzheimer's Disease*. Chicago: Heinemann Library, 2004.

Wilkinson, Beth. *Coping When a Grandparent Has Alzheimer's Disease*. New York: Rosen Publishing Group, Inc., 1992.

INDEX

Published by Creative Education • P.O. Box 227, Mankato, Minnesota 56002
Creative Education is an imprint of The Creative Company
www.thecreativecompany.us
Design and production by The Design Lab • Art direction by Rita Marshall
Printed by Corporate Graphics in the United States of America
Photographs by Alamy (Interfoto, Phototake Inc.), AP Images (Neal Ulevich), Corbis (Bettmann, Michael Freeman), Getty Images (3D Clinic, John Florea/Time & Life Pictures, Hulton Archive, Steve Liss/Time & Life Pictures, MPI, Arnold Newman, Tomohiro Ohsumi/Bloomberg, Zephyr/SPL), iStockphoto (Sebastian Kaulitzki, Duncan Walker); p. 27 illustration © 2011 Etienne Delessert
Copyright © 2012 Creative Education
International copyright reserved in all countries. No part of this book may be reproduced in any form without written permission from the publisher.
Library of Congress Cataloging-in-Publication Data
McAuliffe, Bill. Alzheimer's disease / by Bill McAuliffe. p. cm. — (Living with disease)
Includes bibliographical references and index. Summary: A look at Alzheimer's disease, examining the ways in which it develops, its symptoms and diagnosis, the effects it has on a person's daily life, and research toward finding better treatments.
ISBN 978-1-60818-072-1
1. Alzheimer's disease—Juvenile literature. I. Title. II. Series.
RC523.3.M33 2011   616.8'31—dc22   2010030362

CPSIA: 110310 PO1384
First Edition 9 8 7 6 5 4 3 2 1